Chemotherapy

A Comprehensive Guide to Understanding and Coping with Cancer Treatment

By

Dr. Elizabeth M Harris

TABLE OF CONTENT

INTRODUCTION TO CHEMOTHERAPY

I can confidently claim that it is the severe health issues maintained throughout life. She exhibited no symptoms.

Exactly one year ago, my mother-in-law's 90(a window for 30yrs -veg) was necessary for surgery on the transverse colon. So all blood tests performed on landing at the hospital were confirmed to be regular and adequate. Even after the operation beyond eight months (during standard oral chemotherapy), all the blood tests proved to be expected with no adverse side symptoms via nausea, vomiting, diarrhea etc. She did not lose much hair loss discoloring her hands, as advised.

Chemotherapy is a cancer treatment that employs chemicals to destroy cancer cells. It may be administered alone or with other surgeries or radiation therapy. Chemotherapy interferes with the cancer cell's capacity to grow and divide. It may also help reduce tumors and alleviate pain caused by cancer.

Chemotherapy medications may be administered orally or intravenously, and the treatment plan varies based on the type of cancer being treated. Common adverse effects of chemotherapy include tiredness, nausea, hair loss, and increased risk of infection.

There are different forms of chemotherapy, including combination chemotherapy, adjuvant chemotherapy, neoadjuvant chemotherapy, and more. The choice of chemotherapy medications and treatment strategy is influenced by the kind and stage of cancer and the patient's general health and medical history.

It's crucial to know that chemotherapy is not a cure for cancer but rather a tool to assist in managing and controlling it. Some malignancies may be removed with chemotherapy, while others may only be ordered for a set time.

Chemotherapy may be a very successful treatment choice for many forms of cancer, including breast cancer, lung cancer, leukemia, and others. It is also used to treat cancer that has spread to other places of the body (metastatic cancer) (metastatic cancer).

Patients need to have an open and honest conversation with their healthcare provider about their treatment choices, side effects, and concerns. The healthcare team may collaborate with the patient to establish a treatment plan that suits their particular requirements and objectives.

CHAPTER 1

Definition of chemotherapy

Chemotherapy, usually known as chemo, is a cancer treatment method that includes using chemicals to eradicate cancer cells. The medications target fast-proliferating cells, which is why they are effective against cancer cells.

The chemotherapy medications may be delivered via a vein (intravenously) or in tablet form, and they act by interfering with the cancer cell's capacity to grow and divide. This finally leads to their death.

Chemotherapy is commonly used in combination with other cancer therapies, such as surgery or radiation therapy, to maximize its efficacy and improve results for the patient. The choice of chemotherapy medications and the precise treatment plan will depend on numerous aspects, including the kind and stage of the disease, the patient's general health and medical history, and unique objectives and preferences.

Chemotherapy may be a very successful treatment choice for many forms of cancer and is often used to treat malignancies such as breast cancer, lung cancer, ovarian cancer, and leukemia, among others. It may reduce tumors, ease symptoms, and enhance the chances of cure.

However, it's crucial to understand that chemotherapy may also have adverse effects, including tiredness, nausea, hair loss, and a higher risk of infection. These adverse effects might vary based on the exact medications taken, the dose, and the individual patient. The healthcare team may work with the patient to control these adverse effects and enhance their quality of life.

In certain circumstances, chemotherapy may not be the best therapeutic choice for a patient, and other therapies may be sought. For example, some individuals with early-stage malignancies may need surgery or radiation treatment.

PURPOSE

Chemotherapy aims to destroy cancer cells and reduce tumors. Chemotherapy is commonly used in conjunction with other cancer therapies, such as surgery or radiation therapy, to maximize its efficacy and improve results for the patient.

There are various ways that chemotherapy may aid in the treatment of cancer:

1. **Curative intent:** In certain situations, chemotherapy might be administered as a primary treatment to cure cancer. This is most typically encountered in early-stage malignancies or blood tumors like leukemia.
2. **Adjuvant therapy:** Chemotherapy may be given after surgery to eliminate any leftover cancer cells that may have spread from the initial location.
3. **Neoadjuvant therapy:** In certain circumstances, chemotherapy may be administered before surgery to decrease a giant tumor and make it simpler to remove.
4. **Palliative care:** Chemotherapy may also be used to ease symptoms caused by cancer, such as pain or trouble breathing, and enhance the quality of life for patients with advanced or incurable malignancies.

Types of Chemotherapy

There are various forms of chemotherapy, including:

1. **Combination chemo:** This kind of chemotherapy employs two or more medications simultaneously. The medicines are picked for their positive effects and are meant to boost the overall efficacy of the therapy.
2. **Adjuvant chemotherapy:** Adjuvant chemotherapy is administered after surgery to reduce the likelihood of cancer returning. It is frequently administered to patients with early-stage malignancies to eliminate any leftover cancer cells that may have migrated from the originating location.

3. **Neoadjuvant chemotherapy**: is administered before surgery to reduce a giant tumor, making removing it more straightforward. It may also help lower the likelihood of cancer returning after surgery.

4. **Consolidation chemotherapy:** Consolidation chemotherapy is used after induction chemotherapy to help prevent cancer from coming back.

5. **Maintenance chemotherapy:** Maintenance chemotherapy is used to help protect cancer from coming back following previous therapies, such as surgery or radiation therapy.

6. **Metronomic chemotherapy:** This kind of chemotherapy employs low dosages of medications over a lengthy period to help prevent the disease from developing and spreading.

The choice of chemotherapy medications and treatment plan will depend on the kind and stage of cancer, the patient's general health and medical history, and the patient's particular objectives and preferences.

CHAPTER 2

How Chemotherapy Works

Chemotherapy works by killing or reducing the development of down-regulating cancer cells. Cancer cells grow and divide faster than normal cells, and chemotherapy targets these rapidly developing cells. The medications used in chemotherapy interfere with the DNA and RNA inside the cells, stopping them from dividing and growing.

There are many modes of action for chemotherapeutic medicines, including:

Mechanisms of Action

Chemotherapy medications function by targeting specific pathways that are involved in the development and division of cancer cells. The particular method of action varies depending on the kind of medication; however, some typical processes include:

1. **Interference with DNA Synthesis:** Some chemotherapy medications interfere with DNA synthesis, which is essential for cells to divide and thrive. These medications may prevent cancer cells from reproducing and developing by inhibiting DNA synthesis.
2. **Disruption of microtubules:** Microtubules are structures inside cells that help maintain their form and aid in cell division. Certain chemotherapy medications, such as taxanes, disrupt the microtubules, which may hinder the separation of chromosomes during cell division and lead to cell death.
3. **Inhibition of cell division:** Some chemotherapy medications, such as vinca alkaloids, interfere with the process of cell division by altering the operation of the mitotic spindle, which is essential for cells to divide.
4. **Interference with cell metabolism:** Some chemotherapy medications, such as methotrexate, interfere with the metabolic processes essential for cell growth and division. The medicines may prevent cancer cells from dividing and developing by interrupting these processes.

5. **Induction of apoptosis:** Apoptosis is a natural process of cell death that helps to remove damaged or defective cells. Certain chemotherapy medicines, such as anthracyclines, trigger apoptosis in cancer cells.

These modes of action might differ based on the kind of medicine and the type of cancer being treated. By studying the precise mechanisms of action for each medication, physicians may pick the best suitable chemotherapy treatments for a given patient and cancer type.

Drug Delivery

Chemotherapy medications may be given to the body by numerous techniques, including:

1. **Oral:** Some chemotherapy medications may be administered orally as tablets or capsules. This is the most convenient way of delivery since the patient may take the medicines at home.
2. **Intravenous (IV) infusion:** Many chemotherapy medications are given into the body by an IV infusion. The medicines are usually injected by a vein in the arm or hand and may take several hours to finish.
3. **Intramuscular (IM) injection:** Some chemotherapy medications are given into the muscle, often the upper arm or thigh, using an IM injection.
4. **Subcutaneous injection:** Some chemotherapy medications may be given into the subcutaneous tissue, the layer of tissue under the skin, using a subcutaneous injection.
5. **Intraperitoneal (IP) infusion:** Some chemotherapy medications may be administered directly into the peritoneal cavity, the space inside the abdominal cavity, by an IP infusion.
6. **Topical application:** In rare situations, chemotherapy medications may be administered directly to the skin or mucous membranes.

The distribution method relies on various aspects, including the type of cancer treated, and the patient's general condition. The amount and timing of chemotherapy treatments might also vary based on the patient and the kind of cancer being treated. In general, chemotherapy is often provided in cycles, with a time of treatment followed by a rest period to enable the body to recuperate. This cycle may be repeated numerous times, depending on the patient's reaction to therapy and general health.

Dosage and Timing

The amount and timing of chemotherapy vary depending on various variables, including:

1. **Type of cancer:** The type of cancer being treated might impact the recommended dose and timing of chemotherapy. For example, certain malignancies may need a larger dosage of chemotherapy medications, while others may require a lesser amount
2. **Type of chemotherapy drug:** Varied chemotherapy medications have different suggested doses and regimens. The recommended amount and schedule will depend on the medicine taken, the patient's general health, and other considerations.
3. **Patient's general health:** The patient's overall health, including any existing medical illnesses and therapies, might impact the recommended dose and timing of chemotherapy. For example, a patient with liver or renal disease may need a lower dosage of chemotherapy.
4. **Response to treatment:** The patient's response to treatment will also impact the amount and timing of chemotherapy. If the patient responds well to therapy, the same dose and regimen may be maintained. If the patient is not responding well, the oncologist may alter the amount, schedule, or switch to a different chemotherapy treatment.

<h1 style="text-align:center">CHAPTER 3</h1>

Preparing for Chemotherapy

Preparing for chemotherapy may promote a more accessible and more effective treatment experience. Patients should contact their oncologist about the precise preparatory measures that are advised for their unique treatment; however, some basic actions that might be useful for patients include:

Consultation with Doctor

A consultation with a doctor is a critical stage in the chemotherapy procedure. During the consultation, the doctor will analyze the patient's general health and medical history and the kind and background of the cancer being treated. This information will assist the doctor in selecting the most suitable chemotherapy treatment strategy for the patient.

During the meeting, the patient should share any questions or concerns regarding the therapy, including possible side effects and the impact on their everyday life. The doctor may also offer information on potential advantages and hazards of the medicine and assist the patient in understanding what to expect throughout treatment.

The patient must be fully educated and comfortable with their treatment plan before commencing chemotherapy. If the patient does not understand or agree with any components of the treatment plan, they should address them with their doctor before starting therapy.

Testing and Evaluation

Testing and assessment are crucial components of the chemotherapy procedure. These tests assist the healthcare team in evaluating the kind and stage of cancer, assess the patient's general health and readiness for chemotherapy, and monitor the patient's reaction to treatment. Some frequent tests and assessments done in chemotherapy include:

1. **Diagnostic testing:** These tests assist in diagnosing cancer and define the stage of the illness. Tests may include biopsies, imaging tests (such as CT scans, MRI, and PET scans), and blood tests.
2. **Baseline testing:** Baseline tests, including as complete blood count (CBC), electrolyte levels, and liver and kidney function tests, are conducted before the commencement of chemotherapy to examine the patient's general health and detect any possible concerns that might compromise the treatment.
3. **Monitoring tests:** Monitoring tests are conducted routinely throughout the treatment to evaluate the patient's response to chemotherapy and monitor for any possible adverse effects. Tests may include CBC, liver and kidney function studies, and imaging tests.
4. **Tumor marker testing:** Tumor marker tests are blood tests that evaluate the amounts of certain blood chemicals generated by cancer cells. These tests may help assess the response to therapy and identify the recurrence of the malignancy.
5. **Toxicity testing:** Toxicity tests are conducted routinely throughout treatment to check for any possible adverse effects from the chemotherapy medications. These tests may include liver and kidney function testing and nerve and heart function tests.

The findings of these tests and assessments will assist the healthcare team in deciding the correct dose and timing of the chemotherapy and changing the treatment plan as required. By routinely evaluating the patient's health and reaction to therapy, the healthcare team can ensure the best possible result for the patient.

Chemotherapy

Planning for Treatment

Planning for chemotherapy treatment requires numerous key stages to guarantee the best potential result for the patient. The planning process generally comprises the following steps:

1. **Consultation with the oncologist:** During the consultation, the doctor will analyze the patient's general health, medical history, and the kind and stage of the cancer being treated. This information will help the doctor establish the most suitable chemotherapy treatment strategy.

2. **Development of a treatment plan:** Based on the patient's health situation, the kind and stage of cancer, and the doctor's evaluation, a tailored treatment plan will be produced. This plan will include the type and dose of chemotherapy medications, the frequency and length of treatment, and any additional therapies that may be required (such as surgery, radiation therapy, or immunotherapy) (such as surgery, radiation therapy, or immunotherapy).

3. **Review of probable adverse effects:** The patient should address potential side effects of chemotherapy with their doctor. These may include nausea, vomiting, hair loss, exhaustion, and changes in the patient's skin and nails. The doctor may advise on managing these side effects and what to anticipate throughout treatment.

4. **Preparation for therapy:** The patient should address any questions or concerns with their doctor and healthcare team, and prepare for transportation and support throughout treatment. They may also need to modify their regular schedule to accommodate therapy, such as taking time off from work or curtailing other activities.

5. **Monitoring and follow-up:** During treatment, the patient will have frequent monitoring and follow-up sessions with their doctor and healthcare team. These appointments are essential for monitoring the patient's response to treatment, assessing for side effects, and adjusting the treatment plan.

By working closely with their healthcare team, patients can ensure that they receive the best possible care and support during the chemotherapy treatment process.

CHAPTER 4

Side Effects of Chemotherapy

Chemotherapy is a potent cancer treatment, but it may also induce several adverse effects. The negative effects of chemotherapy might vary based on the kind of medications used, the patient's general health, and the stage of the illness being treated.

Common Side Effects

Common side effects of chemotherapy include:

1. **Nausea and vomiting** are frequent side effects that might develop quickly after chemotherapy treatment and can linger for a few hours to several days. Anti-nausea drugs are commonly recommended to address these symptoms.
2. **Weariness:** Chemotherapy may produce severe fatigue, making it difficult for patients to carry out their everyday tasks. Relaxation may help relieve this adverse effect.
3. **Hair loss:** Hair loss is a typical side effect of chemotherapy, which may include loss of hair on the head, face, and body. This adverse effect is generally transitory, and hair will return after therapy.
4. **Mouth sores:** Chemotherapy may produce sores and a burning feeling in the mouth, making it difficult to eat or drink. The doctor may prescribe drugs to assist in reducing these symptoms.
5. **Skin changes:** Chemotherapy may produce changes in the skin, including dryness, irritation, and discolouration. Keeping the skin hydrated and sheltered from the sun might help control these harmful effects.

6. **Low blood cell counts:** chemotherapy medicines may alter the generation of red and white blood cells, leading to an increased risk of infections and bleeding. Regular blood tests will be conducted throughout therapy to check these levels.

7. **Neuropathy:** Chemotherapy may induce nerve damage, resulting in tingling, numbness, and discomfort in the hands and feet.

8. **Diarrhea:** Chemotherapy may produce diarrhea, which can be treated with dietary adjustments and medicines.

These are some of the most frequent adverse effects of chemotherapy; however the precise side effects a patient may suffer may vary on the kind of medications used, the patient's general health, and the stage of the disease being treated.

Managing Side Effects

Managing the side effects of chemotherapy may help enhance the quality of life for people receiving treatment. Some approaches to control the harmful effects of chemotherapy include:

1. **Drugs:** Anti-nausea medications may help lessen nausea and vomiting, while painkillers can assist in alleviating nerve pain and other discomforts.

2. Lifestyle changes:

3. Eating a balanced diet.

4. Participating in physical exercise.

Obtaining appropriate rest and sleep may help manage tiredness and improve overall health.

1. **Skin care:** Keeping the skin hydrated and shielded from the sun may help prevent skin dryness and discolouration.

2. **Mouth care:** Rinsing the mouth with salt water and avoiding irritants, such as alcohol and spicy meals, will help decrease mouth sores.

3. **Hair protection:** Wearing a hat or scarf to shield the scalp from the sun and avoiding harsh chemicals and heat will help decrease hair loss and stimulate regeneration.

4. **Support:** Joining an assistance group or seeking the support of friends and family may help decrease stress and enhance mental health throughout treatment.

5. **Communication with the healthcare team:** Open communication with the healthcare team may assist in controlling side effects by changing treatment plans and making appropriate modifications to drugs and doses.

It's crucial to communicate to the doctor about any side effects encountered during chemotherapy treatment, as they may propose techniques for controlling these symptoms and assist in enhancing the patient's quality of life throughout treatment.

Coping with Physical Changes

Coping with bodily changes following chemotherapy may be challenging for some individuals. Some ways of dealing with physical changes include:

1. **Acceptance:** Accepting that physical changes may occur throughout chemotherapy and are transient may help alleviate stress and enhance mental health.

2. **Self-care:** Practicing self-care, such as taking frequent breaks, participating in physical exercise, and getting adequate rest, may assist in improving overall health and decreasing stress.

3. **Image support:** Wearing a wig or scarf to disguise hair loss or applying cosmetics to enhance the look of skin changes may assist in increasing self-confidence and decreasing stress.

4. **Support groups:** Joining a support group with other individuals through chemotherapy may create a feeling of community and make patients feel less alienated.

5. **Communication with the healthcare team:** Open communication with the healthcare team may help patients understand the physical changes they are experiencing and establish methods for dealing with them.

6. **Professional counselling:** Talking to a counsellor or therapist may help patients manage stress and enhance mental health throughout treatment.

It's crucial to remember that everyone's experience with chemotherapy is unique, and what works for one person may not work for another. Seeking support from family, friends, and healthcare professionals may help patients deal with physical changes and enhance their quality of life throughout treatment.

CHAPTER 4

Combination Chemotherapy

Combination chemotherapy is a therapeutic method that combines two or more chemotherapy medicines at the same time. The purpose of combination chemotherapy is to maximize the efficiency of the treatment while decreasing the amount of each therapy, which may assist in lessening the severity of side effects. There are various distinct ways that chemotherapy medications may be mixed, including:

Multi-Drug Therapy

Multi-drug therapy, commonly known as polychemotherapy A Guide to a Fit and Healthy Lifestyle", is a therapeutic method that employs numerous chemotherapy medications to treat cancer. The purpose of multi-drug therapy is to maximize the efficacy of the treatment while decreasing the amount of each particular medicine, which may assist in lessening the severity of adverse effects. There are various distinct ways that chemotherapy medications may be mixed in multi-drug treatment, including:

1. Diverse medications with different mechanisms of action: Combining treatments with varying agents might boost the odds of eliminating cancer cells.
2. Pharmaceuticals with positive actions: Combining drugs that function together in various ways may boost the efficacy of the therapy.
3. Treatments that target distinct phases of cell development: Combining drugs targeting different cell growth stages may boost the odds of preventing cancer cells from proliferating and spreading.
4. Pharmaceuticals that have varying toxicities: Combining drugs with distinct toxicities may assist in lessening the severity of side effects by reducing the dosage of each drug.

The choice of medications and the timetable for giving multi-drug treatment is adapted to the individual requirements of each patient. The doctor will examine aspects such as the kind and stage of cancer, the patient's general health, and reaction to prior therapies before deciding on a multi-drug therapy program.

It's crucial to remember that multi-drug therapy may have more significant side effects than single-drug chemotherapy, so patients should consider the risks and advantages of this method with their doctor before commencing treatment.

Targeted Therapy

Targeted therapy is a form of cancer treatment that selectively targets the molecular and genetic abnormalities that cause the development and spread of cancer cells. Unlike typical chemotherapy, which destroys rapidly proliferating cells throughout the body, targeted treatment concentrates on particular chemicals or proteins crucial in cancer cell proliferation and survival.

There are various forms of targeted therapy, including:

1. **Monoclonal antibodies** are laboratory-made proteins that replicate the immune system's capacity to combat illness. They are meant to attach to certain chemicals on cancer cells and prevent their growth or stimulate the immune system to attack the cancer cells.
2. **Small molecule inhibitors are medications** meant to target particular enzymes or proteins involved in the development and survival of cancer cells. They function by stopping the activity of these chemicals and preventing cancer cell development.
3. **Hormone therapies:** These medications target hormones that stimulate the development of particular malignancies, such as breast and prostate tumors.
4. **Immune checkpoint inhibitors:** These medications take the brakes off the immune system, enabling it to target cancer cells more efficiently.

Targeted therapy is typically used with other treatments, such as chemotherapy, radiation therapy, or surgery. It may also be used as a first-line therapy for some forms of cancer, such as chronic myeloid leukemia or certain types of lung cancer.

The use of targeted treatment is customized to the individual requirements of each patient, taking into consideration the kind and stage of cancer and the patient's general condition. Patients should explore the risks and advantages of targeted therapy with their doctor before commencing treatment.

Immunotherapy

Immunotherapy is a cancer treatment that harnesses the strength of the patient's immune system to combat cancer. Immunotherapy aims to assist the immune system in detecting and fighting cancer cells by activating the immune system or directly targeting particular chemicals involved in cancer cell development and survival.

There are various forms of Immunotherapy, including:

1. **Monoclonal antibodies** are laboratory-made proteins that replicate the immune system's capacity to combat illness. They are meant to attach to certain chemicals on cancer cells and prevent their growth or stimulate the immune system to attack the cancer cells.
2. **T-cell therapies** are treatments that employ genetically engineered T-cells, a kind of immune cell, to target and destroy cancer cells.
3. **Cancer vaccines:** These medicines assist the immune system in detecting and fighting cancer cells by exposing them to cancer antigens, which are particular proteins in cancer cells.
4. **Immune checkpoint inhibitors:** These medications take the brakes off the immune system, enabling it to target cancer cells more efficiently.

Immunotherapy is typically used with other therapies, such as chemotherapy, radiation therapy, or surgery. It may also be used as a first-line therapy for some forms of cancer, such as melanoma or certain types of lung cancer.

Immunotherapy is adjusted to the individual requirements of each patient, taking into consideration the kind and stage of cancer and the patient's general condition. Patients should explore the risks and advantages of Immunotherapy with their doctor before commencing treatment.

Chemotherapy and Cancer Staging

Cancer staging refers to identifying the degree to which cancer has spread in the body. Staging helps decide the optimal course of treatment, including chemotherapy.

Chemotherapy is typically used in conjunction with other therapies, like surgery or radiation therapy, to produce the best potential result. The cancer stage may impact the choice of chemotherapy medications, the number of treatment cycles, and the total treatment strategy.

For example, chemotherapy may be taken after surgery in early-stage malignancies to lower the likelihood of the disease returning. In more advanced tumors, chemotherapy may be administered to reduce the tumor before surgery or radiation treatment. In advanced malignancies, chemotherapy may halt the illness's course and enhance the patient's quality of life.

The use of chemotherapy in cancer treatment is adjusted to the individual requirements of each patient, taking into consideration the kind and stage of cancer and the patient's general condition. Patients should examine the risks and advantages of chemotherapy with their doctor before commencing treatment.

Staging of Cancer

Cancer staging identifies the degree to which cancer has spread in the body. The cancer stage helps to decide the right course of therapy and offers critical information about a patient's prognosis.

Cancer staging systems differ based on the kind of cancer but usually incorporate the following factors:

1. **Tumor size and location:** The size and location of the original tumor might give vital information regarding the cancer stage.
2. **Spread to lymph nodes:** The presence or absence of cancer in the adjacent lymph nodes helps to assess whether cancer has spread beyond the primary location.
3. **Spread to other areas of the body:** This information helps to identify whether cancer has spread to distant sections of the body, such as the liver, bones, or lungs.
4. **Grade of the tumor:** The quality of the tumor refers to how abnormal the cancer cells look under a microscope. Higher-grade tumors are more aggressive and have a poorer prognosis than lower-grade tumors.

It's important to note that cancer staging is a dynamic process and can change as treatment progresses and more information becomes available. Patients should discuss the stage of their cancer and its ramifications with their doctor to thoroughly understand their diagnosis and treatment choices.

Chemotherapy for Different Stages

The usage of chemotherapy for various stages of cancer might vary based on the kind of cancer, the set of the illness, and the patient's general condition.

For early-stage tumors, chemotherapy may be taken following surgery to lower the chance of the disease returning. In more advanced tumors, chemotherapy may be administered to reduce the tumor before surgery or radiation treatment. In advanced malignancies, chemotherapy may halt the illness's course and enhance the patient's quality of life.

In certain circumstances, chemotherapy may be used with other therapies, such as surgery, radiation therapy, or Immunotherapy. The precise treatment plan for each patient is adapted to their unique requirements and depends on the stage and kind of cancer and the patient's general condition.

Patients should consider chemotherapy with their doctor for their specific stage of cancer. They may give additional information about the possible advantages and hazards of chemotherapy and assist in establishing a treatment plan that is optimal for the patient.

Alternative Treatment Options

Alternative treatment options to chemotherapy include:

1. **Radiation therapy:** Using high-energy radiation to shrink or destroy cancer cells.
2. **Surgery:** Removing the cancerous tissue through an operation.
3. **Hormonal therapy:** Using drugs or other substances to change the levels of hormones in the body, making it harder for cancer cells to grow.
4. **Immunotherapy:** Using drugs or other substances to stimulate the body's immune system to fight cancer.
5. **Stem cell transplant:** Replacing damaged or destroyed bone marrow with healthy stem cells.
6. **Photodynamic therapy:** Using a special light and a photosensitizing agent to destroy cancer cells.
7. **Palliative care:** Providing comfort and support to patients who have advanced cancer and are not seeking curative treatment.

These alternative treatments may be used alone or in combination with chemotherapy, depending on the stage and type of cancer and the patient's overall health. Patients should discuss their treatment options with their doctor to determine the best course of action for their individual need.

CHAPTER 5

Chemotherapy and Quality of Life

Chemotherapy may have a substantial influence on a person's quality of life. Some typical side effects of chemotherapy, including exhaustion, nausea, and hair loss, might impede a person's ability to carry out regular tasks. However, many people can manage these adverse effects with correct assistance and therapy.

In certain situations, chemotherapy may enhance a person's quality of life by diminishing or halting the course of cancer, lowering pain and other symptoms, and increasing the patient's general well-being. Patients may try to control the harmful effects of chemotherapy and preserve their quality of life. These stages may include:

1. Eating a nutritious diet and keeping hydrated
2. Getting regular exercise
3. Practicing stress-reduction practices, such as meditation or yoga
4. Getting lots of rest and sleep

Talking to a support network, such as family and friends, or a counsellor

Patients should speak to their doctor about the possible impact of chemotherapy on their quality of life and discuss measures to control any side effects that may emerge during treatment.

Impact on Daily Life

Chemotherapy may have a substantial influence on everyday living. Some typical side effects, such as tiredness, nausea, and hair loss, might make it challenging to carry out routine tasks. However, many people can manage these adverse effects with correct assistance and therapy.

In certain situations, chemotherapy may also enhance everyday life by diminishing or halting the course of the disease, lowering pain and other symptoms, and improving the patient's general well-being. Patients may take precautions to reduce the effect of chemotherapy on their everyday lives.

These stages may include:

1. Planning for treatment and rehabilitation time, including taking time off from work or modifying work hours
2. Making alterations to the home environment, such as building handrails or changing furniture to make it simpler to move about
3. Seeking assistance from family and friends or joining a support group for cancer patients
4. Practice self-care, such as eating a good diet, regularly exercising, and obtaining enough rest and sleep.

It's vital for patients to speak to their doctor about the possible effect of chemotherapy on their everyday life and to express any concerns they may have. The doctor can give guidance and tools to assist patients in handling any issues they may face throughout treatment.

Support Systems

Having a solid support system is a crucial element of dealing with chemotherapy. Family and friends may give emotional support, assist with home responsibilities, and provide transportation to and from treatments. Other sorts of assistance that may be useful for patients include:

1. **Cancer support groups:** These groups give a venue for sufferers to discuss their experiences and provide one other emotional support.

2. **Counselling:** Talking to a competent counsellor may help patients handle the stress and emotions that typically accompany a cancer diagnosis and treatment.
3. **Complementary therapies:** Therapies such as acupuncture, massage, and meditation may help reduce stress and enhance general well-being.
4. **Support from healthcare providers:** Patients should feel comfortable talking to their doctor, nurse, or other healthcare practitioners about their experiences and any worries they may have.

Patients should seek their support network for aid and support whenever they need it. It's also crucial for patients to be proactive in seeking assistance and services that may help them handle chemotherapy's physical, emotional, and practical problems.

Managing Emotional Distress

Chemotherapy may be a challenging and stressful experience, and it's usual for patients to suffer emotions of grief, worry, and dread. Here are some techniques to assist in minimizing mental discomfort during chemotherapy:

1. **Talk to a mental health professional:** Talking to a therapist or counsellor may help people process their feelings and develop techniques to manage stress and worry.
2. **Join a support group:** Support groups bring together individuals experiencing similar issues, and they may give a feeling of community and a space to discuss experiences and emotions.
3. **Practice self-care:** Engaging in activities that provide pleasure and relaxation, such as exercise, hobbies, or spending time with loved ones, may help decrease stress and increase overall well-being.
4. **Stay connected with loved ones:** Spending time with friends and family, or clicking with those who have gone through similar circumstances, may bring comfort and support.
5. **Keep a journal:** Writing down thoughts and feelings may help patients manage their emotions and bring a sense of relief.

It's vital to remember that it's natural to feel overwhelmed and nervous at times and that these emotions do not represent a lack of strength or bravery. Patients should speak to their doctor or a mental health expert if they feel their feelings harm their ability to handle day-to-day tasks.

CONCLUSION

Chemotherapy is a cancer treatment that employs chemicals to eliminate cancer cells. It is a frequent treatment for many forms of cancer and may be used alone or in conjunction with other therapies, such as radiation therapy or surgery.

Chemotherapy may have a range of adverse effects, including nausea, exhaustion, and hair loss. However, medicine or lifestyle adjustments may frequently address these negative effects.

Patients must have a robust support system and seek services to assist in handling the physical, mental, and practical problems of chemotherapy. Patients should also be proactive in discussing their treatment choices with their doctor and asking questions about their concerns.

Summary of Key Points:

Chemotherapy is a cancer treatment method that employs chemicals to eliminate cancer cells. It may be used alone or with other radiation therapy or surgical therapies. Chemotherapy may have a range of adverse effects, including nausea, exhaustion, and hair loss. It is crucial to have a solid support system and seek out tools to handle chemotherapy's physical, emotional, and logistical problems. Patients should be proactive in discussing their treatment choices with their doctor and asking questions about their concerns.

Continuing care is a vital component of the process after completing chemotherapy treatment. It needs regular monitoring and cares to ensure cancer does not return and to manage any possible long-term complications of the therapy.

Continuing treatment may include frequent check-ups with a doctor, imaging tests to monitor cancer, and physical and psychological help to handle any residual side effects or emotional discomfort.

Patients who have taken chemotherapy are at increased risk for specific health issues, such as heart disease, osteoporosis, and infertility; thus, it is vital for them to be aware of these possible dangers and to make efforts to control them.

It is crucial for patients to engage closely with their healthcare team and to be proactive in seeking out services and help when required. This may guarantee the best possible results and a seamless transition to life following chemotherapy.

Future research in the area of chemotherapy will continue to concentrate on enhancing the efficacy and lowering the harmful effects of the treatment. This may entail creating novel medications and combination therapies, enhancing delivery techniques, and better understanding the processes through which chemotherapeutic agents function.

There is also a rising emphasis on personalized medicine in chemotherapy, with researchers studying the use of genetic and molecular profiling to customize treatment to each patient's particular requirements and features.

Researchers will continue exploring the long-term consequences of chemotherapy, focusing on enhancing survivors' quality of life and identifying strategies to manage and avoid long-term health issues connected with the treatment.